LEAK NO MORE

What your parents never told you about good bladder and bowel habits

---

2nd Edition, Revised and Expanded

BY

DR. NATALIE PADVEEN PT, DPT

Leak No More

TABLE OF CONTENTS

Leak No More

INTRODUCTION

I originally published this book just over two years ago. However, I decided that a revision was warranted due to all the evidence-based science and information that continues to come out. I decided to write this book because, as a pelvic health physical therapist, my biggest frustration when meeting new patients is the lack of education about their bladder and bowel health that they received when they were younger. Early education about good or healthy bladder and bowel habits could prevent suffering, embarrassment, and expense later in life. Twenty-five million adults suffer from urinary incontinence, and 75-80% of those people are women (Wu et al., 2014). We also know that the incidence of pelvic floor dysfunction increases with age. Urinary incontinence costs US men and women more than $20 billion annually in supplies and medical management (Subak et al., 2008). Because of shame or embarrassment, people continue to suffer in silence.

A common misconception is that pelvic floor dysfunction only affects people who have given birth, but this is not the case. Pelvic floor dysfunction can affect anyone, including children and athletes. People do not realize that they can make minor changes in their daily routine to avoid the occurrence of pelvic floor dysfunction, possibly prevent it, or at least minimize the risk of occurrence. For this reason, I decided to write this book. I hope that the information provided in this book helps bring awareness to this issue so that we can reduce the incidence of pelvic floor dysfunction and save people from additional long-term financial expenses and embarrassment while improving their quality of life.

I believe pelvic health education should be provided at the elementary school level in conjunction with sex education. Interestingly, The National Institute for Health and Care Excellence (NICE) in the UK recently recommended that girls aged 12 to 17 be taught pelvic floor exercises in school, which could help them avoid issues such as incontinence later in life (BBC News, 2021). What a novel idea!

I hope those who read this book use the information garnered to start making lifestyle changes, including training and educating their families and loved ones about good bladder and bowel habits. The sooner we start, the better off we will be.

CHAPTER 1

The Basics

Not being taught about good bladder and bowel habits from an early age can increase your chance of developing pelvic floor dysfunction.

What is the pelvic floor?

The pelvic floor is a complex group of muscles and tissues that support the pelvic organs, including the bladder, uterus, and rectum. The pelvic floor extends from the pubic bone in the front to the tailbone at the back and up both sides of the hip bones. It acts like a sling or a hammock supporting what lies on top, and three layers of muscle form this sling/hammock. Coordinated contraction and relaxation of the pelvic floor muscles control the bowel and bladder functions – the pelvic floor must contract to prevent unwanted leakage and relax to allow for urination, bowel movements, and sexual intercourse. The urethra, where the bladder empties, the vagina, and the anus open and pass through your pelvic floor. The pelvic floor also helps with blood flow to improve orgasm and acts as a sump pump to aid with lymphatic drainage and blood circulation.

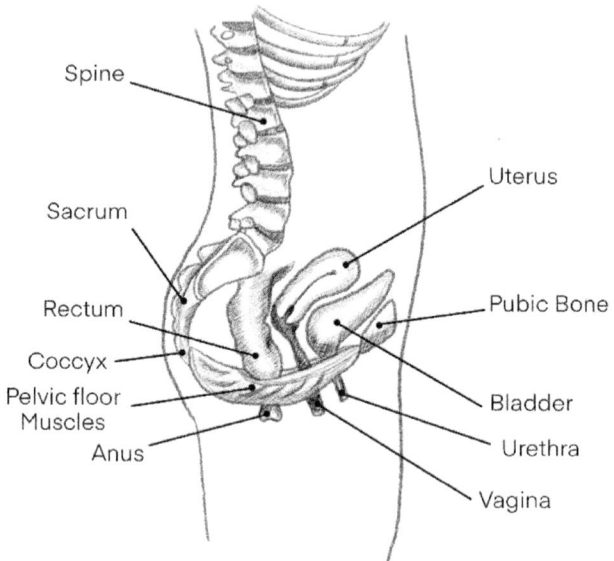

Figure 1. The Pelvic Floor

What is pelvic floor dysfunction?

Pelvic floor dysfunction (PFD) is a term used to describe a problem with the muscles in the pelvis. PFD occurs when there is either too much tension in the pelvic floor muscles or not enough. This often contributes to urinary incontinence, constipation, pain during intercourse, or pain in the lower back, pelvic region, genitals, or rectum.

What are examples of pelvic floor dysfunction?

A pelvic floor dysfunction typically refers to:

1. Urinary incontinence (leakage of urine)
2. Fecal incontinence (leakage of stool)
3. Pelvic Organ Prolapse
4. Pelvic Pain

(In this book, I will focus mainly on the first three problems).

What is the incidence of PFD?

Based on a cross-sectional study of a nationally representative population of women in the United States, the prevalence of at least one type of PFD was 23.7%. The prevalence doubled in women 80 or older (Hallock & Handa, 2016). The probability that a woman will undergo surgical correction of a pelvic organ prolapse by age 80 is estimated to be one in five (Hallock & Handa, 2016). Also, studies show that many women simultaneously suffer from more than one type of pelvic floor dysfunction (Rortveit et al., 2010).

What does the term continence mean?

Continence is the ability to control movements of the bowels and bladder. It is the ability to stay dry or clean.

Urinary incontinence is divided into three categories: *stress*, *urge*, and a combination of both, referred to as *mixed* incontinence. Stress urinary incontinence (SUI) is urine leakage due to increased intra-abdominal pressure that occurs with a cough, sneeze, laughing, or jumping, among other things. When pelvic floor muscles are weak, they cannot withstand the downward pressure placed on them, resulting in leakage of urine, feces, or both.

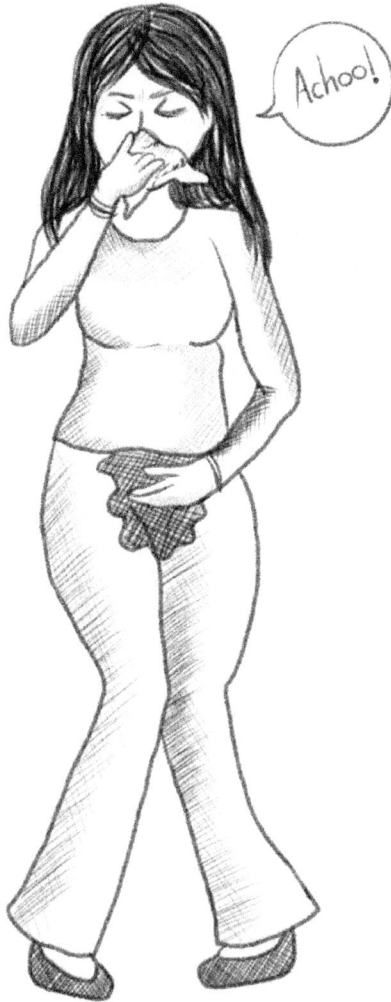

Figure 2. Stress Urinary Incontinence

Urinary urge incontinence (UUI) occurs from poor bladder habits or increased pelvic floor muscle tension. Mixed urinary incontinence (MUI) is a combination of both SUI and UUI.

Fecal incontinence is usually due to urge incontinence, a strong and sudden urge to go to the bathroom where you have a bowel movement before getting to the toilet on time, soiling your underwear. This is more common with a loose stool.

What is a pelvic organ prolapse?

Pelvic organ prolapse (POP) occurs when the tissue and muscles of the pelvic floor can no longer support the pelvic organs, resulting in the drop (prolapse) of the pelvic organs from their normal position. The pelvic organs include the vagina, cervix, uterus, bladder, urethra, and rectum. A prolapse of any of these organs can occur. In the following image (Figure 3), the left picture shows the normal placement of the organs in our bodies. If you look at the bladder, it looks funnel-shaped, allowing the urine in the bladder to empty fully. Now, look at the image of the bladder on the right. Because of muscle weakness or muscle tension, the back wall of the bladder drops down from its proper position, or better said, leans into an area where there is more space, the vaginal canal. This is a bladder prolapse, and urine can get stuck because of the pocket created (see the image of the arrow). Then, when you stand up to walk away, the urine trapped in the pocket can now dribble out as the organs shift.

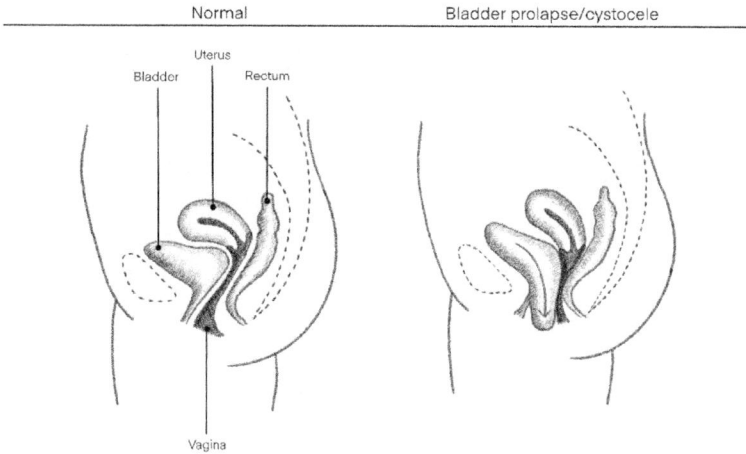

Figure 3. Pelvic Organ Prolapse of the bladder.

POP typically occurs when the pelvic floor muscles become weak or when excessive pressure is applied to the pelvic floor muscles regularly. This can happen with vaginal childbirth or over time with chronic constipation, violent coughing or heavy lifting, or heavy impact activity (even running).

What does having a pelvic organ prolapse feel like?

Many people can have a POP but do not even know they have one. In contrast, others may experience symptoms such as vaginal bulging or bleeding, pelvic pressure or heaviness, low backache, vaginal discharge or more frequent infections, pain with intercourse, needing to splint (use of a finger, thumb, or tool in the vaginal canal) to give support or assist in emptying their bowels, or a worsening of symptoms when gravity is present, or activity is increased. Some people may experience urinary incontinence as a result.

What are the risk factors for developing pelvic floor dysfunction?

Sometimes, pelvic floor dysfunction can be genetic. Some people have weaker muscles and connective tissue, but more often, it results from injuries to the pelvic area. Damage can occur during childbirth and from pelvic surgery. Using the pelvic muscles excessively (like going to the bathroom too often or pushing too hard) eventually leads to poor muscle coordination. Being overweight will often worsen these issues as well as advancing age or getting older. Other factors contributing to pelvic floor dysfunction are heavy lifting or exertion, especially when the breath is held with the activity. This will increase the intraabdominal pressure on the pelvic floor muscles. For a similar reason, chronic constipation can contribute to pelvic floor dysfunction. High-impact activities such as running and jumping or improper exercise form can also lead to issues. People who smoke are at higher risk of developing pelvic organ prolapse because smoking damages connective tissue in our bodies.

Another factor that cannot be fully controlled is menopause. Pelvic floor muscles need estrogen to stay strong, and SUI and POP are more common with the loss of estrogen during menopause. Preparing and keeping a strong pelvic core can reduce the symptoms when this loss of estrogen occurs.

Other less common causes include neurological disease; certain medications can sometimes contribute to incontinence.

Is it only women who develop pelvic floor dysfunctions?

Children can also develop pelvic floor dysfunction. One of the biggest causes of pelvic floor dysfunction in children is constipation. Also, nocturnal enuresis or bed wetting is highly prevalent in children, specifically 5%-10% at age seven and 1%-2% in adolescents (Bogaert et al., 2020).

More than 30% of young gymnasts, with an average age of 14.5, reported issues with SUI (Gram & Bo, 2020).

Men have pelvic floor muscles, too, and can also develop pelvic floor dysfunction. While it does primarily affect women, 16% of men have been identified with PFD (Smith, CP., 2016). Almost 80% of men experience incontinence following prostatectomy, and many are still incontinent 12 months post-surgery (Litwin et al., 2001).

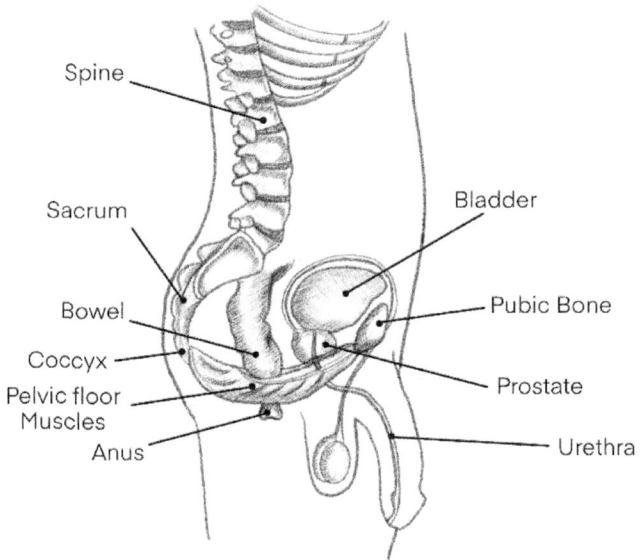

Figure 4. The male anatomy with pelvic floor

Are pelvic floor dysfunctions preventable?

Many causes are preventable or can be reduced unless they are primarily caused by pregnancy, delivering a baby, or pelvic surgery. That is why education is so important. Maintaining lower body weight, avoiding constipation and straining, showing good posture, and using good lifting techniques, such as exhaling with exertion, decrease the risk of developing PFD.

.

CHAPTER 2

Good Bowel Habits to Follow

First, it is essential to maintain good fluid intake. The National Academy of Medicine (2019) suggests an adequate intake of daily fluids of about 13 cups for men and 9 cups for women, with 1 cup equaling 8 ounces. These recommendations cover fluids from water and other drinks and foods such as tea, soup, juice, etc. Usually, about 20% of daily fluid intake comes from food and the rest from drinks.

Fluid intake recommendations are not set in stone. They can and should be adjusted based on your circumstances. If you are working out, you must compensate for the fluid lost from sweating. You will want to drink before, during, and after a workout. If the temperature outside is extremely hot or you are at a high altitude, you will also need to drink more fluid to prevent dehydration. Pregnant or nursing women also need added fluid to stay hydrated as they share their supplies. Lastly, increased fluid intake will be essential to compensate for the fluid loss if you are ill with a temperature or vomiting.

Water is not the only source of fluid. Many fruits and vegetables are composed chiefly of water, such as watermelons, radishes, and cucumbers. Drinks such as milk, juice, and herbal teas are mostly water. Ideally, you should avoid drinks high in sugar, such as soda, as they have minimal health benefits. Also, alcohol dehydrates, so do not include it in your daily total. Surprisingly, coffee can be included in your daily total fluid intake. Even though we consider coffee a bladder irritant, which we will discuss in the next chapter, it is not a diuretic and will not contribute to dehydration (Grandjean et al., 2000).

How do you know if you are drinking enough water?

Observing the color of your urine is a fantastic way to determine if you are drinking enough water. If it is dark, you are most likely not consuming enough—the more transparent the color, the less yellow, the better.

The following chart is a good fluid intake guideline to start with. As you can see, the amount differs by age.

AGE	DAILY ADEQUATE INTAKE
1-3 years	4 cups, or 32 ounces
4-8 years	5 cups, or 40 ounces
9-13 years	7-8 cups, or 56-64 ounces
14-18 years	8-11 cups, or 64-88 ounces
Women, 19 and older	9 cups, or 72 ounces
Pregnant women	10 cups, or 80 ounces
Breastfeeding women	13 cups, or 104 ounces

National Academy of Medicine, 2019

Figure 5. Water intake chart by age

Why is water important for our bowel health?

When we eat food and drink water, the digestive system converts the food into its simplest form, which is then absorbed into the bloodstream from the small intestine. Nutrients are then carried to each cell in the body.

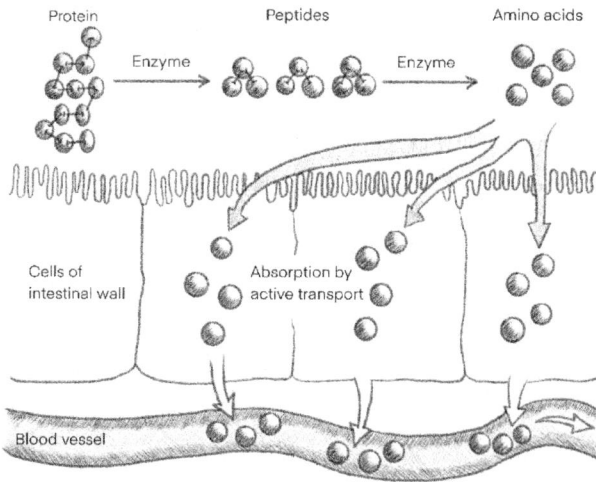

Figure 6. What occurs at the cellular level?

Our large intestine plays a key role here. Its job is to absorb the remaining water and other nutrients from the indigestible material, solidifying it to make stool. So, if you do not drink enough water, and your body absorbs water back into your bloodstream, your stool will most likely become hard, dry, and difficult to expel, causing constipation.

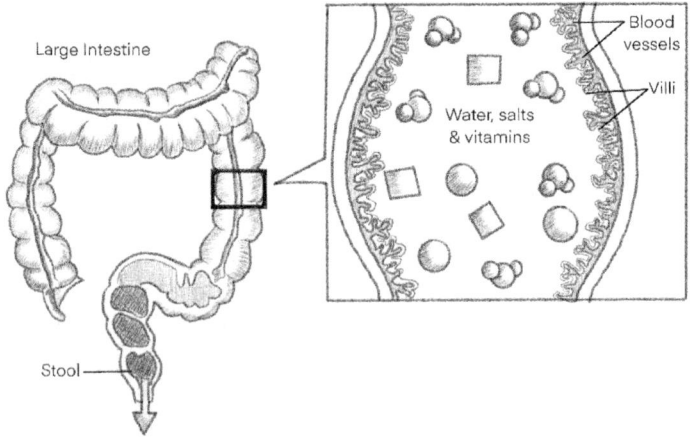

Figure 7. Water is reabsorbed in the descending colon

Constipation leads to the need to strain to have a bowel movement. Chronic straining increases intraabdominal downward pressure on the pelvic floor, weakening it and predisposing it to develop pelvic floor dysfunction. So, keeping a good fluid intake will help prevent constipation.

How do you know if you are constipated?

You are constipated if you have fewer than three bowel movements a week and your stool is hard, dry, and difficult to pass. In addition to increasing our water intake, we also need to increase our **fiber** intake. Fiber is found in plant-based foods. We do not digest fiber. It passes through the stomach, intestines, and colon and then out of the body. There are two types of dietary fiber: soluble fiber – found mainly in fruits and vegetables – and insoluble fiber, primarily in cereals and whole grains. Soluble dietary fibers help soften stool in the body, and insoluble fibers help bulk stool, making it easier to empty with less bearing down or straining.

How much fiber do we need?

The requirement for fiber varies with age. Kranz et al. (2012) supplied a table of fiber requirements for various age groups:

Children 1 to 3 years: 19 grams of fiber/day
Children 4 to 8 years: 25 grams of fiber/day
Boys 9 to 13 years: 31 grams of fiber/day
Girls 9 to 13 years: 26 grams of fiber/day
Boys 14 to 19 years: 38 grams of fiber/day
Girls 14 to 19 years: 26 grams of fiber/day

According to the U.S. government's 2015 Dietary Guidelines, women should **eat at least 21 to 25 grams of fiber daily**, while **men should aim for 30 to 38 grams daily.**

It should be noted that these are only general guidelines. Please check with your primary care physician to confirm how much fiber you should consume before making dietary changes.

If you increase your fiber intake, do it slowly. As mentioned previously, you must also increase your water intake. Not drinking enough water contributes to constipation (Chung et al., 1999).

So, what foods can you eat that are high in fiber?

The following is a rudimentary list to help get you going. Still, it is best to consult with a registered dietician and gastroenterologist if you are struggling with constipation or other GI issues.

High-Fiber Food List (see the following four pages)

Source: USDA National Nutrient Database for Standard Reference, Legacy Release

Vegetables	Serving size	Total fiber (grams)*
Green peas, boiled	1 cup	9.0
Broccoli, boiled	1 cup chopped	5.0
Turnip greens, boiled	1 cup	5.0
Brussels sprouts, boiled	1 cup	4.0
Potato, with skin, baked	1 medium	4.0
Sweet corn, boiled	1 cup	3.5
Cauliflower, raw	1 cup chopped	2.0
Carrot, raw	1 medium	1.5

Fruits	Serving size	Total fiber (grams)*
Raspberries	1 cup	8.0
Pear	1 medium	5.5
Apple, with skin	1 medium	4.5
Banana	1 medium	3.0
Orange	1 medium	3.0
Strawberries	1 cup	3.0

Grains	Serving size	Total fiber (grams)*
Spaghetti, whole-wheat, cooked	1 cup	6.0
Barley, pearled, cooked	1 cup	6.0
Bran flakes	3/4 cup	5.5
Quinoa, cooked	1 cup	5.0
Oat bran muffin	1 medium	5.0
Oatmeal, instant, cooked	1 cup	5.0
Popcorn, air-popped	3 cups	3.5
Brown rice, cooked	1 cup	3.5
Bread, whole-wheat	1 slice	2.0
Bread, rye	1 slice	2.0

Leak No More

Legumes, nuts and seeds	Serving size	Total fiber (grams)*
Split peas, boiled	1 cup	16.0
Lentils, boiled	1 cup	15.5
Black beans, boiled	1 cup	15.0
Baked beans, canned	1 cup	10.0
Chia seeds	1 ounce	10.0
Almonds	1 ounce (23 nuts)	3.5
Pistachios	1 ounce (49 nuts)	3.0
Sunflower kernels	1 ounce	3.0

*Rounded to the nearest 0.5 gram.

For more information on food fiber content, I recommend visiting www.nutrition.va.gov.

What foods should we avoid if we are constipated?

- Foods that are low in fiber and high in fat.
- Frozen and processed foods are high in sodium and thus absorb water needed for digestion from your large intestines, resulting in harder dry stool. Also, processed foods are low in fiber; for example, white rice, which is brown rice stripped of wheat, germ, and husks, is lower in fiber. One cup of brown rice has 3.5 grams of fiber, while one cup of white rice has only 1.42 grams.
- Stay well hydrated. As previously mentioned, dehydration or not drinking enough water will worsen constipation.
- Avoid red meat as it is harder to digest.
- Un-ripened bananas are more constipating than ripe ones.
- People with gluten sensitivity should do well to avoid gluten as this can worsen constipation.

Does fiber have other health benefits?

- Fiber helps lower cholesterol levels (Brown et al., 1999).
- Fiber helps control blood sugar levels (Anderson et al., 2009).
- Fiber aids in achieving and keeping a healthy weight (Miketinas et al., 2019).
- Fiber helps you live longer (Reynolds et al., 2019).

What other tips can you share?

When you feel the urge to have a bowel movement (BM), do not wait!

Holding in stool for too long often messes with our natural defecatory [bowel movement (BM)] reflexes. So, if possible, go within 10 minutes of feeling the urge to have a BM. If you fear public toilets, make a nest of toilet paper and sit. Squatting or hovering over a toilet seat to have a BM engages our pelvic floor muscles, making it harder to pass the stool. When sitting, do not strain! Allow your belly to expand and think, "Belly big, belly hard," which engages the abdominal muscles and creates a 'safe' amount of intraabdominal pressure.

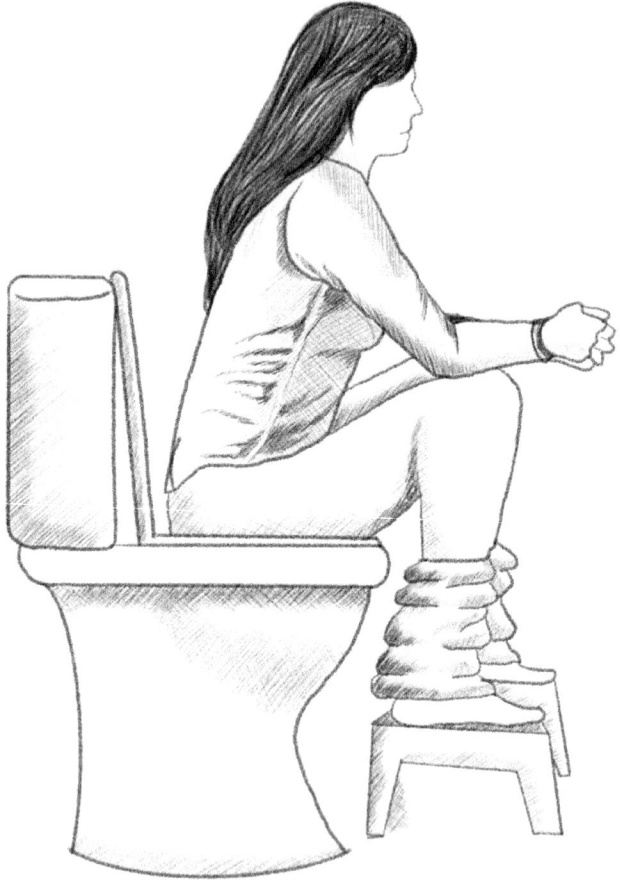

Figure 8. Good toileting posture

If possible, place your feet on a stool so your knees are higher than your hips, and rest your forearms on your thighs, as this helps widen the recto-anal angle through which the stool needs to pass. Vocalizing or making a sound with your mouth helps, too. Please do not be shy; let it out! The sound is "MOOOOOO." Think "MOO" to "POO." If you are having trouble with bowel movements, try again later. You do not want to sit on the toilet for too long as it can cause more problems with your pelvic floor. Ideally, limit your sitting time to 5 minutes.

Are you not feeling the urge yet? Get up and move. Walking helps trigger peristalsis, which is the involuntary movement of the muscles of our intestines, aiding the forward movement of its contents. A regular walking plan, even 10 to 15 minutes several times a day, can help the body and digestive system work at their best.

You should always use a step stool or "squatty potty" for peeing and when having a bowel movement, and most importantly, you should NEVER hover over a toilet seat.

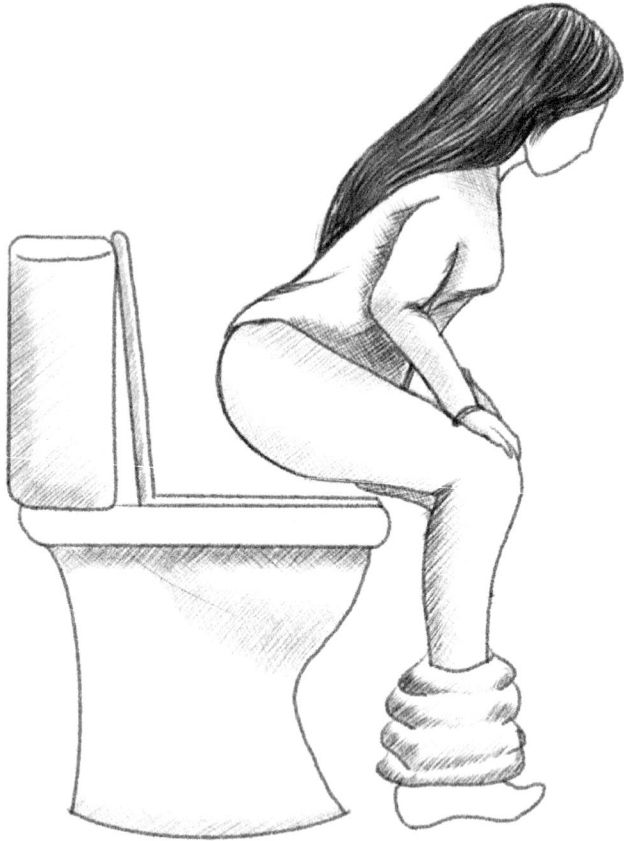

Figure 9. Squatting or hovering over the toilet seat

Hovering causes you to contract or engage your pelvic floor muscles, which is the last thing you want to do when you are trying to pee or poo. Think of it this way. When you walk around throughout the day, urine and stool are not leaking out (ideally) because our pelvic floor muscles are engaged. Our brain instructs our pelvic floor to contract its muscles to keep everything inside. When you sit at your desk, your brain recognizes that you are sitting on a chair, not a toilet, so your muscles stay engaged or contracted so you do not soil the chair. When you sit on a toilet seat, your brain recognizes that it is now time to pee or poo, so your pelvic floor muscles should relax to empty your bladder or rectum fully. So, if you are hovering because you are afraid of germs on a toilet seat, your brain gets confused and does not know if it should relax or contract because you are neither sitting nor standing. Because the muscles are not relaxed, you need to force the urine out or strain, which creates increased downward pressure on the pelvic floor muscles, weakening them. Hovering often will weaken and damage your pelvic floor muscles, so sit!

Leak No More

CHAPTER 3

Good Bladder Habits to Follow

You've seen the commercials where a woman is franticly saying, "got to go, got to go, got to go!"

People who experience urinary urgency and frequency, also known as an overactive bladder, feel a sudden urge to pee and will often leak before making it to the toilet. Sometimes certain medications we take can cause this, so speak to your doctor to rule that out. Other times, it could be due to poor bladder habits or tight pelvic floor muscles. Tight pelvic floor muscles can put pressure on the urethra and bladder, making you feel like you must go to the bathroom or as though you did not fully empty your bladder and you still need to go, but these signals can be controlled.

There is a reflex between the bladder and the pelvic floor muscles. This reflex works by allowing the pelvic floor muscles to relax when it is time to pee and the bladder contracts, and the opposite, ensuring the pelvic floor muscles are engaged when the bladder is relaxed, and it is not time to go. We can use this reflex to help control urgency and prevent leakage.

You must perform the following urge suppression techniques to control these urgent signals.

a. **Be still/stop moving.** When you experience this strong urge, stop moving. If you can, sit down, as applying pressure to the perineum (the opening of the vagina) inhibits (or stops) the bladder from contracting. Sometimes, if you are flexible enough, sitting on your heel helps, too. Even though it may sound counterintuitive, rushing to the bathroom increases anxiety and the sympathetic input to the bladder, leading to leakage, so do not rush.

b. **Perform Quick Pelvic Floor Muscle Contractions.** Once you have stopped moving or are sitting down, perform 4-5 quick and small pelvic floor muscle contractions to use the reflex between the pelvic floor and the bladder. (How to correctly contract your pelvic floor muscles will be addressed in Chapter 4.) Typically, the pelvic floor will relax so the bladder can empty, but if we start to contract our pelvic floor muscles, this will signal the bladder that it is not yet time to empty, helping reduce the urge.

c. **360-Degree Deep Breathing.** After performing 4-5 pelvic floor contractions, slowly inhale through your nose and think of filling a balloon in the lower part of your abdomen. As you inhale through your nose, allow the lower ribs to expand outward in all directions, like an umbrella opening. Then, slowly deflate the balloon by blowing out your mouth like you are blowing out candles. Repeat this 4-5 times slowly and calmly. This slow breath work decreases the sympathetic input to the bladder and helps with the sense of urgency. For a more thorough description of how to perform this breath work, refer to page 38.

d. **Distraction.** Lastly, do whatever it takes to distract your mind from the bathroom. You can count backward from 100 by 7's or 20 by 3's. Visualize a favorite time or place, or use self-talk, "I am in control," while performing 360-degree deep breathing, etc. Get creative!

What is considered a normal voiding (bladder emptying) interval?

Average urine output is 6-8 times per day or every 3-4 hours. As we age, we may need to pass urine more often, but no more than every two hours, so if you are peeing more often, use the earlier urge suppression techniques to hold off going to the bathroom. Start with a smaller goal to be successful; maybe start holding off for an hour and a half, and as you notice improvement, increase the interval by which you are holding off by an additional fifteen minutes each week until you get to that three-hour interval. If you can use these techniques successfully, have held off for three hours, and still feel an urge, then calmly walk to the restroom to pee. If you rush, you risk the chance of leakage. If the urge creeps up again as you walk towards the bathroom, repeat your urge suppression techniques before walking into the bathroom until you can calmly walk to the toilet, slowly lower your pants, and calmly sit without leakage. You may need to keep a chair or stool right outside your bathroom for such cases to calm down and collect yourself before entering the restroom.

Interestingly, **just like peeing too often, it is possible not to go often enough. You want to avoid consistently ignoring the urge to go to the bathroom for longer than 4 hours.** This can lead to other problems that this book will not address.

Remember that a suitable time interval for peeing is between 2 and 4 hours.

Can anything else contribute to my urinary urgency?

Not drinking enough water or ingesting bladder irritants can contribute to urinary urgency. Have you ever rinsed your mouth with Listerine mouthwash? Usually, you cannot keep it in your mouth for too long because it burns. The lining of our mouth is the same as the lining of our bladder, so just like mouthwash, urine that is too concentrated because you are not drinking enough water can function as a bladder irritant. So, increasing your water intake can dilute your urine and make it less irritating to the bladder. Certain foods and drinks can also function as bladder irritants.

Common examples of bladder irritants are:

- Caffeine – coffee, tea
- Carbonated drinks, including carbonated water.
- Alcohol – wine, beer, etc.
- Artificial sweetener
- Chocolate
- Smoking
- Citrus fruit and juices
- Tomato and tomato-based products.
- Spicy food

If you notice an increase in urinary urgency after ingesting any of the above items, try cutting them out of your diet and see if that influences your symptoms. Ultimately, that may be the culprit.

Is there anything else I could be doing that is contributing to bad bladder habits?

Avoid or stop going to the bathroom *"just in case."* This is a tough one. I am unsure about you, but I have been trained to go to the bathroom whenever I leave my house. I grew up in Canada, and whenever I wanted to play outside in the snow, my parents made me go to the bathroom before putting on my snowsuit. They were never taught that this could contribute to urinary urgency and frequency! So, if you have a problem with urinary urgency, you need to STOP going to the bathroom "just in case." For example, if you voided (peed) 45 minutes ago and are leaving to meet a friend for dinner, do not use the restroom before leaving your house. Use your urge suppression techniques to hold off the urge if it presents, and calmly walk to the closest available restroom when the time is right (2 hours after the last time you peed). It may be challenging in the beginning, but it is possible. You will be so happy you did not give up and stuck with it.

What if a tight pelvic floor is the main cause of my urinary urgency?

If you have a tight pelvic floor or are unsure what is causing your urinary urgency, you should visit a pelvic floor physical therapist near you for more guidance. You will want to avoid doing "Kegels" or pelvic floor muscle contractions as this can exacerbate or worsen your symptoms. Your goal will be to relax your pelvic floor muscles, and one way to do so is through 360-degree deep breathing. Yoga, gentle stretching, mindfulness, and meditation are great ways to relax the pelvic floor. Women who suffer from pelvic pain should focus on these techniques as tight pelvic floor muscles are often, but not always, the cause.

How do I do 360-degree deep breathing?

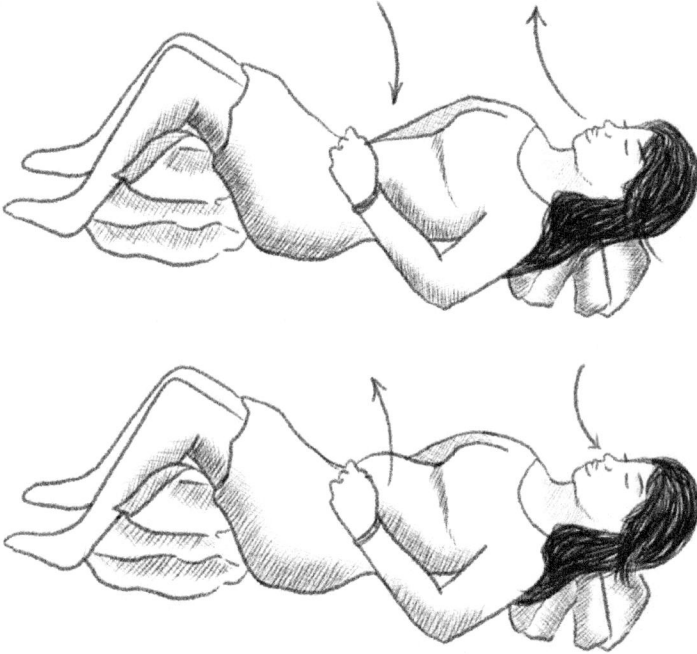

Figure 10. 360-degree deep breathing

It was briefly described as part of the urge suppression techniques, but here it is in more detail.

360-degree deep breathing can be done in any position. Place one hand on your lower belly and the other on your chest. Imagine that there is a balloon under the belly hand. As you inhale through your nose, direct the air to the balloon in the belly so it gently inflates. Do not strain or bear down. Ideally, the belly and chest hand will rise evenly, but the air should not go into your neck or shoulders. There should be equal expansion throughout the lower ribs into the back, belly, sides, and chest. It should be a relaxed inhalation. Then, to 'deflate' the balloon, blow out your mouth as if you are blowing out a candle. Take slow and calming breaths and continue to breathe like this for 3-5 minutes, gradually taking longer breaths, keeping them smooth and slow.

This method of breathing will do two things. First, it will stimulate your parasympathetic nervous system to promote a state of calmness. Second, its piston-like action with the other body organs, including your lungs and diaphragm, will promote lengthening of the pelvic floor muscles. Consider deep breathing as stretching muscles you cannot see, such as your pelvic floor muscles.

Are there any other times I should be doing this 360-degree deep breathing?

You just learned that this breathing style is an excellent way to relax and lengthen or stretch the pelvic floor muscles. As we have often been taught, it is essential always to stretch before and after exercise, so if you do not have any issues with increased pelvic floor muscle tension but do experience muscle weakness resulting in urinary or fecal incontinence or pelvic organ prolapse, you will want to strengthen your pelvic floor muscles by performing strengthening exercises. Like any exercise, you will always want to stretch before and after exercising. 360-degree deep breathing is how we "stretch" our pelvic floor muscles before and after performing pelvic floor muscle strengthening exercises.

CHAPTER 4

Pelvic Floor and Core Muscle Training

Who should exercise their pelvic floor muscles?

As I mentioned in the earlier chapter, if you have pelvic pain, you will want to avoid pelvic floor muscle training. Not forever, but until you can fully relax your pelvic floor muscles and no longer experience pain.

If you suffer from stress urinary incontinence or pelvic organ prolapse and have been cleared to exercise by a pelvic health therapist, you will want to strengthen your pelvic floor. Studies show that pelvic floor muscle training can improve symptoms of urinary incontinence and significantly improve the quality of life in most people (Curillo-Aguirre et al., 2023).

How do you perform pelvic floor strengthening exercises?

For some people, this can be very tricky and sometimes frustrating. Not everyone has the coordination to perform a pelvic floor contraction correctly, otherwise known as a "Kegel."

One helpful cue often used is to "Imagine you are trying to slow the urine flow." It is important to remember that you are not doing this when sitting on the toilet seat because, as previously said when we sit on the toilet, the brain recognizes that it is time to relax the muscles and empty the bladder. If we try to slow the urine flow when sitting on the toilet, we will weaken the muscles we are trying to strengthen. So, please understand that this technique is only used to help visualize slowing the flow of urine and should not be done while urinating. When we envision slowing the flow of urine instead of stopping it, it will be easier to activate the pelvic floor muscles without activating the glutes and abdominal muscles. Initially, we want to isolate the pelvic floor muscles without engaging other muscles. Once you can do this, you will eventually add larger muscle groups to your training program.

Here are helpful cues that may help if you have a vagina:

- Think of "nodding your clitoris."
- Imagine you are trying to stop the passing of gas.
- Imagine a zipper running from your vagina to your pubic bone. Now consider closing that zipper.
- Imagine you are sucking up a thick vanilla milkshake through a straw at the vaginal opening.
- Try to draw your tailbone towards your pubic bone to pick up a marble.

Common cues that are helpful if you have a penis:

- Imagine you are trying to shorten your penis.
- Think "Nuts to guts."
- Try to lift your scrotum.

Interestingly, we all have two types of muscle fibers in our pelvic floor muscles, just like in all the muscles in our body, and these need to be trained differently. Just like marathon runners and sprinters train differently, we need to strengthen our pelvic floor muscles using two strengthening exercises. **Remember**, before starting, we always want to stretch, so perform 2-3 minutes of deep breathing to relax the muscles before you move on to strengthening.

It is essential to understand that you cannot strengthen a tight muscle, so to attain optimal length, you will want to relax the muscles before beginning your exercises. To explain this more clearly, imagine you are doing a bicep curl.

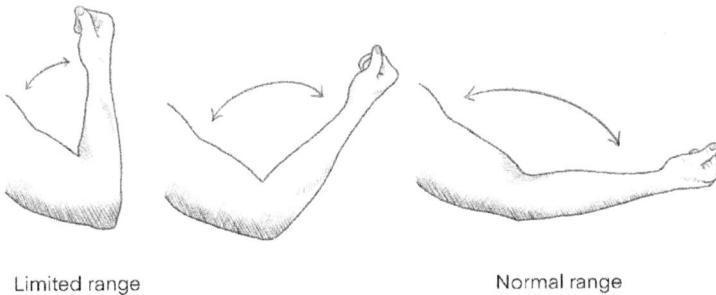

Limited range

Normal range

Figure 11. Elbow range of motion

If you have a healthy elbow and can fully extend and bend your elbow, you can strengthen your bicep through its full range of motion. However, if you injure your elbow and cannot straighten it all the way, you cannot strengthen it through its full range of motion, so the muscle will weaken. If you carry tension in your pelvic floor, you must relax and lengthen the muscles before strengthening them to maximize your workout.

The slow-twitch, endurance, marathon-runner-type muscle fibers in our pelvic floor hold our organs up all day or enable us to hold off voiding until we reach a bathroom that may not be readily accessible. We use our breath to help strengthen these, and we will review how that works in the next section.

The fast twitch, sprinter-type explosive muscle fibers found in our pelvic floor prevent leakage when there is a strong increase in downward pressure, such as during a strong cough or sneeze. When strengthening these muscles, you should be able to breathe normally and even converse while performing pelvic floor contractions. Nobody should be able to tell what you are up to.

How do you strengthen your pelvic floor muscles for endurance?

After 2-3 minutes of 360-degree deep breathing, you will first inhale and let your belly and lower rib cage expand equally. Then, upon exhalation, engage your pelvic floor using the visual cues supplied earlier (page 42), holding the contraction for 5 seconds. Then, inhale and relax the pelvic floor for 5 seconds. Repeat this process ten times.

How do you strengthen your pelvic floor muscles for power and speed?

The count for this exercise is a 2-count to contract the pelvic floor and a 2-count to relax the pelvic floor, and it should be repeated ten times. Remember that you want your muscles to work through their full range of motion rather than rachet up and tighten. The tempo is "contract 1, 2" and "relax 1, 2." It takes two seconds to contract your pelvic floor and two seconds to relax fully. Do not squeeze your glutes or other muscles; breathe naturally. There should not be any sign that you are exercising. When practicing these, it may be helpful to place your hands on your glutes; if you feel your glutes contract, you are not doing them correctly.

Remember always to finish your exercises with deep breathing to ensure your muscles return to full length and are ready to work when needed, such as when coughing, sneezing, or laughing. You do not want to leak because your muscles are tight from exercising.

To Recap:

1. **Perform 2-3 minutes of 360-degree deep breathing.**
2. **Work the marathon runners or perform slow contractions using your breath to help. Inhale to relax the muscles, and then upon exhalation, contract your pelvic floor muscles for 5 seconds, inhale, and relax for 5 seconds. Repeat ten times.**
3. **Work the sprinters (aka Quick Flicks). While breathing normally, contract for two counts and relax for two counts. Repeat ten times.**
4. **Always finish with 360-degree deep breathing for 2-3 minutes.**

Frequency: This whole series 3x/day

Will I have to do these forever?

Yes! Like any muscle, **you lose it if you do not use it!** Make your pelvic floor exercises part of your daily routine. If you brush your teeth after every meal, then do these exercises after you brush your teeth! The only time you should stop is if the exercises cause pain. If you experience pain, see your medical provider.

Are there any other common-sense tips I should know?

Practice doing a pelvic floor contraction just before you perform an activity that typically causes you to leak. For example, if you feel a sneeze coming on, in the time it takes to reach out and grab a tissue, you should already be engaging your pelvic floor in preparation for the intense downward pressure. Think, "Squeeze before you sneeze." In physical therapy, we call this performing "the knack." You may also want to use "the knack" when lifting something heavy or when you laugh or cough.

Another tip is never to hold your breath or strain upon exertion, as this causes an increase in intraabdominal pressure, which damages the pelvic floor. Remember to always **exhale on exertion** when lifting or pushing. Whether lifting your baby's car seat, moving a sofa across the room, or lifting weights at the gym, you always want to exhale on exertion or think, "Blow as you go."

Lastly, knowing that your pelvic floor is a crucial part of your core is essential. When discussing the core, we often think of the 'abs' or the 'six pack.' However, the core is more than just that. It includes the transverse abdominis, the deepest abdominal muscles on the front side of the body, the multifidus muscles of the spine, the breathing diaphragm up top, and the pelvic floor muscles at the base. Understanding this can help you appreciate the role of your pelvic floor in your overall health and wellness.

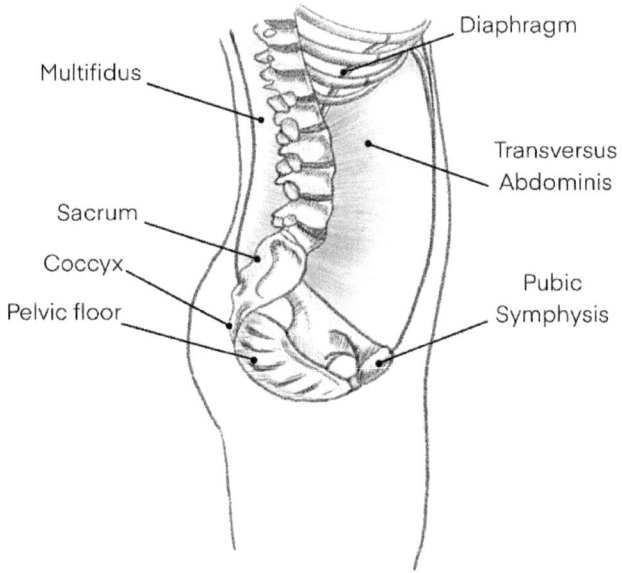

Figure 12. The core

How do I engage my core?

All these muscles work together to stabilize the spine, creating a sturdy support base. Without this sturdy base, injury and dysfunction can occur. When looking for an exercise program, finding an integrated approach to strengthen the whole 'pelvic core' is essential as this will lead to more benefits than "Kegels" alone. Interestingly, you cannot activate your transverse abdominis (the deepest of the abdominal wall muscles) without activating your pelvic floor. They work together. Many people do not know how to engage their core correctly, so here are some tips:

- While lying on your back with your knees bent, place your fingers on top of your hip bones and then move them about an inch closer to your midline so that the pads of your fingers rest on the area just inside the hip bones.

- While breathing normally, gently draw your belly button towards your spine and ribs down towards your belly button (they should not flare out).

- Lastly, make what I call an "angry librarian" noise. **SH!** Make this quick sound while ensuring your belly stays drawn in. If your belly pushes out when you say **SH!** you are doing it wrong.

- Can you keep this engagement and continue to breathe normally while exercising?

With your core engaged correctly, you should be able to do different exercises with your arms and legs without losing this engagement. If you lose the engagement of your deep core muscles, stop the exercise and reset before continuing. It takes practice, but once you know how to connect with those deep core muscles, you will feel stronger and safer with any workout routine.

CHAPTER 5

Pelvic Floor Strengthening & Improved Sexual Functioning

As mentioned in earlier chapters, those who do not have pelvic pain can and should work on pelvic strengthening exercises.

Not only does pelvic core strengthening decrease lower back pain and urinary incontinence and help build muscular endurance, but it can also be highly beneficial to people's sex lives.

How can pelvic floor training and strengthening improve sex?

- A strong pelvic floor can boost arousal, increase blood flow, intensify orgasms, and improve sexual relations and intimacy (Lowenstein et al., 2010).

- Pelvic floor muscle training can help increase blood flow to the pelvic area, reducing dryness and genitourinary symptoms of menopause (GSM), which can result in heightened sensitivity and arousal (Mercier et al., 2016).

- Pelvic floor exercises performed after giving birth help "tighten" the vaginal area making intercourse more pleasurable (Kolberg-Tennfjord, 2015).

- In women, more blood flow to the clitoris and vagina, with pelvic floor training means that those areas will be more sensitive and intensify sensations and orgasm (Sartori et al., 2021). In men, strengthening the pelvic floor muscles can improve sexual function, such as erections, orgasms, and ejaculations (Cohen et al., 2016).

- Research has suggested that women who regularly do proper pelvic exercises are more likely to experience vaginal orgasms. Women who do these exercises report more intense orgasms and more frequent orgasms (Kanter et al., 2015).

- Pelvic floor muscle strengthening exercises boost libido and improve orgasm (Kizilkaya et al., 2003).

- Pelvic floor training in post-menopausal women helps reduce pelvic floor dysfunction (Franco et al., 2021). Pelvic exercises can give women more confidence in their sexuality, bodies, and sexual performance.

CHAPTER 6

Good Vulvar Care and Hygiene

Most people think that washing that area with plain old soap and water is the best solution, but the vulvar tissue or skin is extremely sensitive and easily irritated. Typical items that can irritate the tissue are bodily fluids, including urine, feces, and sweat; feminine or baby wipes, shampoos, and soaps; perfumed toilet paper; tight clothing, sweaty clothing; clothing washed in certain detergents or fabric softeners; nylon underwear or synthetic undergarments; spermicides and other chemicals, even tea tree oil.

So, how are you supposed to wash down there?

I typically tell my patients to treat their vulva like a self-cleaning oven and only use warm water when washing.

If you insist on using a cleanser to clean yourself, use an unscented, non-alkaline cleanser such as Cetaphil or a mild soap for sensitive skin such as Dove or Neutrogena. Also, avoid rubbing the vulva. Ideally, soak for five minutes in lukewarm water to remove sweat or residue, and gently pat the area dry.

Is there anything else I should be doing?

Yes, if you work out or sweat a lot, change out of your sweaty clothes as soon as possible. White cotton underwear is best, although it is not always the prettiest. Stay away from bubble baths and avoid feminine hygiene sprays. Do not use wipes, and only use white, unscented toilet paper. Remember, do not rub, but pat yourself dry. Lastly, when doing laundry, use a mild, hypoallergenic laundry detergent, like the ones people use to wash baby clothing, and avoid fabric softeners.

CHAPTER 7

Pregnancy and Beyond

Unfortunately, one of the most common occurrences that happen later in pregnancy, especially as our growing bellies place more downward pressure on our bladders, is that we develop stress urinary incontinence (SUI). This often occurs with sneezing, laughing, coughing, jumping, exercising, and bending. This is not something to stress over (pardon the pun), as studies show that 18-75 % of pregnant women experience it (Rajavuori et al., 2021), especially in their third trimester. Another study found that the prevalence of SUI was 11% in the first trimester, 50% in the third trimester, and 16.4% at six months postpartum (Molinet et al., 2022), proving that it does improve. During pregnancy, our bodies experience a surge in the relaxin hormone. The ovaries and the placenta produce this hormone to prepare a woman's body for childbirth. It relaxes the ligaments in the pelvis and softens and widens the cervix. As a result of the relaxation of the tissue in our pelvis and our growing bellies, there is little support for our bladder, which worsens urinary leakage.

What are the risk factors for developing SUI during pregnancy?

- Older age
- Being overweight
- Having a previous vaginal delivery

- Having previous pelvic surgery

- Smoking, which we learned weakens our connective tissue and can often result in chronic coughing, increasing the intraabdominal pressure placed on the pelvic floor muscles.

Since weight gain contributes to stress urinary incontinence, moderate daily exercise will help you maintain a healthy weight. Confirm with your doctor before starting any new exercise program, and make sure there is no reason for your doctor to recommend against it.

We also know pelvic trauma during delivery can contribute to stress urinary incontinence (SUI), pelvic organ prolapse (POP), and pain after delivery. Perineal massage to stretch the perineum, the opening of the vagina, in the weeks before delivery has been shown to reduce the risk of tearing or needing an episiotomy (Beckmann & Garrett, 2006) and, therefore, reducing the risk of developing a pelvic floor dysfunction. This can typically be started at 34 weeks of gestation if you do not have any of the following contraindications: *placenta previa, vaginal bleeding, infection such as vaginal herpes or thrush, or are placed on pelvic rest.* To be safe, consult with your medical provider before you begin perineal massage.

How do I do perineal massage?

First, you will want to get into a comfortable position. You can prop yourself on several pillows to support your body and growing belly. Ensure that your legs are supported to relax your pelvic floor muscles better. Then apply a generous amount of water-based lubricant (see the Appendix for lubricant suggestions) to your thumb and insert your thumb about an inch into the vagina. When you do this, your thumb will face downwards, away from your face. You can start with one thumb and eventually use two thumbs. Everyone has different dexterity, different length arms, and different size bellies, making this more challenging for some compared to others. Do not hesitate to ask your partner for help if you have trouble reaching the area. Using one thumb to start, apply gentle downward and outward pressure, moving your thumbs in a U-shaped motion. This will allow you to stretch the vaginal tissue, muscles, and skin of the perineum. You will only need to do this in the tissue that is closest to the anus. If you imagine that the opening of the vagina is a clock, with 12 o'clock where the clitoris is and 6 o'clock at the bottom or back side closest to the anus. 3 o'clock will be on your left and 9 o'clock on your right. The area you want to massage will be between 3 and 9, moving through 6 o'clock, hence a "U" shape. Initially, you may feel burning or stinging, but this should pass as everything loosens. Performing your 360-degree deep breathing helps you relax better during this massage. Ideally, you will want to do this for 5-10 minutes daily or every other day until your baby is born. Be prepared for discomfort, as you will most likely feel an intense burning pain when you begin to stretch. Work each area on the lower half of your "clock," holding the stretch for at least one minute. Work deeper into the stretch as you breathe through it if the tissue begins to relax. When you feel you are not getting enough stretch with one thumb, add a second for a deeper stretch. If you do not have a partner to help you and find it challenging to reach, the ***Frida Mom Prepare-to-push Perineal Massage wand*** can be extremely helpful.

Much research supports using a warm compress applied to the perineum while pushing to reduce the severity of tearing (Magoga, G. 2019). So, speak to your OB to see if they can do this or allow someone else to do this for you.

So, will I stop leaking urine once the baby is born?

The risk for postpartum urine leakage goes up with higher birth weight babies and with the number of babies that a woman has delivered. Typically, bladder control should return to normal after about six weeks, but if you continue to experience issues, see a pelvic health specialist.

When a woman chooses to breastfeed, the body produces prolactin to support a good milk supply, producing less estrogen. Our muscles need estrogen to function optimally. In some women, it takes as long as six months after having stopped nursing for their hormone levels to return to normal (Hormone Health Network, 2018). As a result, nursing women may experience genitourinary symptoms of lactation (GSL), which include vaginal atrophy, vaginal dryness, pain with intercourse, and urinary incontinence (Perelmuter et al., 2024). Often vaginal estrogen is prescribed to lactating mothers to decrease these symptoms.

If you have diastasis rectus abdominis (DRA), a separation of the abdominal muscles, after delivery and you see doming or tenting in the middle of your stomach with specific movements, or you are experiencing symptoms of a POP, such as increased pelvic pressure that worsens at the end of the day, take a breath. As your hormone levels normalize with time, these issues will also improve.

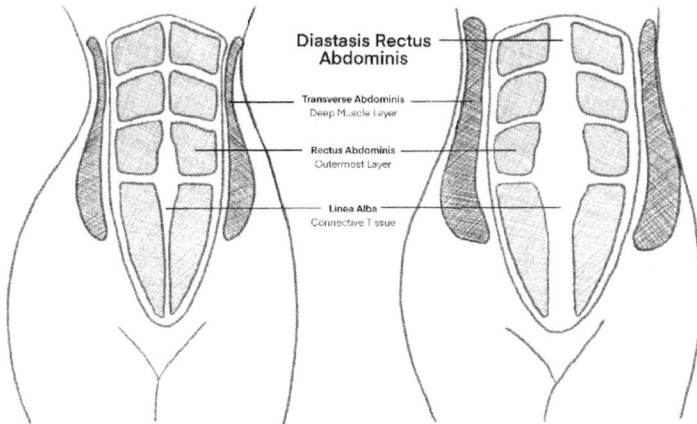

Figure 13. Diastasis Rectus Abdominis

What can I do to help things along?

First, at your 6-week follow-up appointment, ask your OB-gynecologist to refer you to a pelvic health physical therapist. Secondly, watch your body mechanics. When you were pregnant, I can guarantee your body mechanics were not at their best. After 40 weeks of pregnancy, we forget how to move correctly and safely. If you have a DRA and see tenting or coning as you change positions, take it as a sign that you are moving incorrectly. A pelvic health physical therapist can teach you how to reconnect with your deep core muscles to reduce the tenting and prevent DRA from worsening. Incontinence can be managed by performing pelvic floor strengthening exercises, working on weight loss, and following good lifestyle habits.

Ideally, doing all these things before getting pregnant would be best. Doing so can limit or prevent symptoms during pregnancy and make recovery easier following pregnancy.

CHAPTER 8

Menopause, Oh No!

So, here is some not-so-great news. Menopause can wreak havoc on your pelvic floor. As mentioned earlier in this book, our pelvic floor muscles rely on estrogen to support strength and integrity. With menopause, our organs stop producing estrogen, causing our pelvic floor muscles to weaken. However, they do not just weaken; they shrink (or, more accurately, atrophy)!

What pelvic floor issues do postmenopausal women develop?

Postmenopausal women are known to develop what is called genitourinary symptoms of menopause (GSM), which can include:

- Vaginal dryness
- Vaginal burning
- Vaginal discharge
- Genital itching
- Burning with urination
- Urgency with urination
- Recurrent urinary tract infections
- Urinary incontinence
- Light bleeding after intercourse
- Discomfort with intercourse.
- Decreased vaginal lubrication during sexual activity.
- Shortening and tightening of the vaginal canal

A whole book can be written on this topic, and many have been. However, I hope that by reading this book, you can be prepared and prevent these conditions from taking over your life. Urinary incontinence affects more than 50% of postmenopausal women (Kolodynska et al., 2019), and the number of people it affects increases yearly. As already mentioned, urinary incontinence negatively affects all aspects of life, affecting work, physical activity, and sexual health, and urinary incontinence is the main symptom of GSM.

The stronger your pelvic floor is before menopause, the fewer issues you will experience. If you have never done pelvic floor training and are just starting now, do not despair. Chapter 5 research shows that pelvic floor muscle exercises can improve the sexual function of postmenopausal women and are, therefore, suggested to be included in healthcare packages designed for postmenopausal women (Nazarpour et al., 2018). Another study showed pelvic floor muscle training as an effective treatment for postmenopausal women with GSM and urinary incontinence (Mercier et al., 2019). You are never too old to start, but starting young helps.

Women who suffer from GSM are often treated with vaginal estrogen. Vaginal estrogen works locally and is not systemic like hormone replacement therapy (HRT). The type of estrogen prescribed by physicians is typically estradiol, the most potent form of estrogen, and can come in different forms, including creams like Premarin or Estrace, suppositories like Vagifem or Imvexxy, or rings such as Estring. Other treatments that can be helpful include vaginal moisturizers such as Revaree or Good Clean Love, Restore, which do not need a prescription (see appendix).

Another consequence of loss of estrogen in postmenopausal women is recurrent urinary tract infections (UTIs). This occurs because as estrogen levels drop, our good bacteria, Lactobacillus, drops too, and the vaginal pH goes up. Vaginal estrogen improves the vaginal microbiome reducing the prevalence of recurrent UTIs.

Leak No More

CHAPTER 9

What About Surgery?

Often people want a quick fix, but the International Continence Society Guidelines recommend conservative treatment as the first line of treatment for urinary incontinence (Syan & Brucker, 2016) and that surgery should only be considered when conservative treatment will not bring positive results.

What is a conservative treatment for urinary incontinence and pelvic organ prolapse?

Conservative treatment typically includes pelvic therapy, behavioral therapy, and medication. Some medication helps lessen the symptoms of an overactive bladder by reducing the muscle activity in the bladder and, therefore, the sense of urgency. The urge suppression techniques taught in Chapter 3 are examples of behavioral training techniques used by pelvic health physical therapists to treat an overactive bladder. A part of a pelvic physical therapist's job is to work on behavioral training related to the bladder and bowel.

Lifestyle changes, which have been discussed throughout this book, such as weight loss, stopping smoking, breathing correctly with exertion, or managing our internal pressures, including avoiding constipation, are just some of the things that fall into the realm of what pelvic health physical therapists do. Instructing patients on correct exercise forms and the importance of doing these exercises for the rest of their lives are all part of what a pelvic physical therapist will teach their patients.

For stress urinary incontinence, where medication is not effective, pelvic floor muscle training emerges as a highly successful treatment. Numerous studies have consistently shown that this training not only reduces or eliminates urinary incontinence but also alleviates associated depressive symptoms and improves quality of life. Recent reports indicate that a significant 80% of patients who underwent pelvic physical therapy for stress urinary incontinence experienced positive results. When combined with weight loss, pelvic floor muscle training was the most effective conservative treatment for stress urinary incontinence.

An underused conservative treatment for pelvic organ prolapse is the pessary. A pessary, usually made of silicone, is inserted into the vagina to correct vaginal prolapse and, at times, stress urinary incontinence. Pessaries come in various forms and sizes, and your physician or pelvic floor physical therapist can decide which is best for you. They are easily removable, so you can choose when to wear them. You may not need to wear one when sitting all day at work but could benefit from one when going for a run. A pessary is like a bra for your organs. Once you are home for the night, remove your pessary just like you would remove your bra. Both treatment with a pessary and treatment with surgery showed a clinically significant improvement in prolapse symptoms (Van der Vaart, L. et al., 2022), showing the benefits of trying a pessary. The guidelines of the Dutch College of General Practitioners recommend that women with stress urinary incontinence be offered treatment of pelvic floor muscle training and a pessary as initial treatment; a mid-urethral sling (surgery) should only be discussed when initial therapy is insufficient or in the case with severe symptoms (Daman-Van Beek, 2016). Pessaries offer a great alternative, especially for those who are not healthy enough to undergo surgery or are waiting for surgery. Some women will choose to put off having surgery until they know they will not get pregnant again, for it is known that about 50% of women who have a vaginal birth will have some prolapse.

Studies have shown that using a pessary with pelvic floor training reduces prolapse symptoms and improves the quality of life (Cheung et al., 2016). Pessaries help lift the organs off the pelvic floor muscles, making it easier to perform pelvic floor contractions and allow the muscles to work through their full range of motion. The importance of this was discussed in chapter 4.

Another documented benefit of using a pessary is the remodeling of the vaginal tissue. If you think of the pelvic floor muscles as a sling with a hole in the center, and you think of the organ that is dropping down to be a bowling ball, you can imagine that the more the bowling ball presses down on the sling with a hole, the larger the hole will get. This hole in the female body is referred to as the genital hiatus. We have been discussing it in simpler terms, such as the vaginal opening. Women with a prolapsed organ will develop a larger genital hiatus or vaginal opening. However, long-term use of a pessary has been shown to reduce the stage or the distance that the organ drops and the size of the genital hiatus (Boyd et al., 2021). Not only is this great for function, but it is also great for appearance and sexual confidence.

OK, that is all great, but what if I want surgery?

The most common surgeries to treat stress urinary incontinence are performed through an incision (cut) in the abdomen, through the vagina, or with laparoscopy, where smaller incisions are made in the abdomen. According to the American College of Obstetrics and Gynecology (ACOG), surgery aims to lift or support the urethra and the neck of the bladder.

There are two types of surgery to treat pelvic organ prolapse: obliterative and reconstructive. Obliterative surgery narrows or closes off the vagina to provide support for prolapsed organs. Sexual intercourse is not possible after this procedure. Obliterative surgery has a high success rate and may be a desirable choice if you do not plan to have intercourse in the future and want an easily performed procedure (ACOG, 2021). Reconstructive type surgeries include surgeries that aim to return the organs to their original and correct position to reduce or eliminate the symptoms of pelvic organ prolapse. As with any surgery, there are many risks, so talk with your healthcare professional about which option is best for you.

If you choose the surgical route, please ask your surgeon for a referral to a pelvic health physical therapist, not just after surgery but before, too. Studies show that "routine pre and postoperative physiotherapy interventions improve physical outcomes and quality of life in women undergoing corrective surgery for urinary incontinence and pelvic organ prolapse" (Jarvis et al., 2005).

CHAPTER 10

Your New Roll for This Old Issue

Now that you are better informed, you must stop suffering in silence. After reading this book, you should realize that you are not alone and are not the only one dealing with these issues. Usually, when a group of women is out for dinner, and a woman confesses to leaking urine after they have been drinking wine, and someone tells a funny joke, there is a collective sigh of relief, and then everyone starts chattering about how it has happened to them, too. It is funny how we feel we now have 'permission' to discuss our truth. We, indeed, are a sisterhood.

You need to be proactive in sharing all the knowledge you just received. Go onto Facebook, Instagram, and any other social media platforms you use and share, share, share. You can be confident that your information is evidence-based and backed by research. Create your support team. Find a gynecologist, urogynecologist, and pelvic health physical therapist, and surround yourself with a knowledgeable and supportive health team. Do not be afraid to ask questions when you go for routine checkups; if you do not find the answers you want, ask for referrals elsewhere. Today, you should be able to find answers and solutions or alternatives to all your medical needs. Do not settle for anything less. Whether you are preparing to deliver a baby, just had a baby, or are going through menopause, your support team should be there to turn to for all your needs, even as those needs continue to change. And they will.

If you carry a few extra pounds, join a gym, grab a friend or dog, and walk. Just get up and move! In the next chapter, I will summarize the key points you must remember. All the facts will help you achieve your goal of leaking no more. Please make a copy of the next page and keep it as a reminder of what you should or should not be doing. It is easy to revert to old bad habits when life gets busy.

CHAPTER 11

Wrapping It All Up

If you get anything from this book, please remember the following key points.

1. Drink more water!
2. Avoid constipation and increase your fiber intake.
3. When you feel the urge to have a BM, do not delay!
4. Normal voiding intervals for urinating are between 2-4 hours.
5. Do not make it a habit of holding your pee for more than 4 hours.
6. Do not hover over the toilet seat! Sit down!
7. Avoid going to the bathroom 'just in case.'
8. Do not hold your breath. Always exhale on exertion or 'blow as you go.'
9. When sitting on the toilet, whether peeing or having a bowel movement, use a step stool or "squatty potty" so that your knees are higher than your hips. Lean forward and rest your forearms on your thighs. This makes perfect toileting posture.
10. Keep moving! Walk, do yoga, and do anything that you enjoy. Just get up and move!

Bonus tip: Never stop exercising your pelvic floor! If you do not use it, you lose it. Make a routine and do your exercise daily. Yes, for the rest of your life!

Teach your kids good bowel and bladder habits today so they can grow up knowing more than we did and help stop the leakage!

APPENDIX
Lubricant Suggestions

Lubricants are used to reduce friction and are typically applied right before intercourse.

Water-based lubricants are best because they will not increase the risk of an altered microbiome that could lead to bacterial vaginosis, a common vaginal infection. The following are lubricants, with many studies supporting their safety and effectiveness.

- Pre-Seed
- Good Clean Love Biogenesis
- Aloe Cadabra

Some people prefer oil-based lubricants, but it is essential to know that they can cause blockage to the glands in the vulva for some people. Also, oil-based lubricants can damage latex condoms and, as mentioned above, can affect vaginal ph.

Whatever lubricant you choose, you want to ensure it does not contain preservatives, glycerin, petroleum, or warming agents. Other ingredients to avoid include artificial flavors, colors, sugars, and essential oils, which can cause reactions in some people.

Over-the-counter support for POP

If you are unsure whether you want to be fitted for a pessary, the following are some over-the-counter products you could try. If they relieve any or all your symptoms, investing time and money to be properly fitted for a pessary may make sense.

- Impressa -comes in three sizes: single use for 12 hours.
- Revive – one size fits most; it can be used for 31 days but worn for 12 hours.
- Uresta – five sizes to choose from. It lasts for one year but can only be worn 24 hours at a time.

Vaginal Moisturizers

While vaginal lubricants sit on the surface of the skin to make penetration more comfortable, vaginal moisturizers are absorbed by the skin. Moisturizers work to trap and hold moisture in the skin. They are typically used when a person experiences vaginal dryness, as often occurs postpartum and post-menopause, as women are in a low estrogen state. Some over-the-counter examples include:

- Replens
- Ah! Yes Long-Lasting Vaginal Gel Moisturizer
- Kindra Daily Vaginal Lotion and or V Relief Serum

- Revaree by Bonafide

Some people prefer natural or homemade products such as coconut oil, almond oil, olive oil, and vitamin E. However, oil-based products, including food-grade products, can negatively affect vaginal ph.

Hyaluronic acid, a natural substance found in our bodies, has been shown to improve or reduce tissue atrophy, improve cell maturation, vaginal ph., and vaginal symptoms (Dos Santos et al., 2021). The following are examples of moisturizers containing hyaluronic acid:

- Hyalogyn gel

- Revaree by Bonafide

- Good Clean Love

- Gynatrof

Vulvar Balms

Not to make you more confused, balms are another category of topicals that can be used for vaginal dryness. Whereas vaginal moisturizers can be applied both internally and externally, balms are typically applied only externally.

Vulvar balms are formulated to go externally on the vulva (the outside of the vagina), can be applied daily to provide a protective layer, and are often used regardless of estrogen status. Balms are often oil blends that protect the skin's natural acid mantle and maintain proper pH levels. The following are examples of vaginal balms:

- Vmagic Vulva Balm

- Intimate Rose Enchanted Rose Vulvar Balm

- Aquaphor

- Rosebud Woman Honor Vulvar Balm

Vaginal Probiotics

New research is emerging on the use of probiotic capsules used vaginally in the prevention of chronic UTIs (Gupta et al., 2024). *Lactobacillus acidophilus* is the most-researched strain of probiotics when it comes to establishing and maintaining a healthy vaginal biome. Two other essential strains include *lactobacillus rhamnosus* and *lactobacillus reuteri*. Interestingly, vaginal probiotics taken orally can help vaginal odor. You can take some vaginal probiotics orally and insert others as suppositories into your vagina. The following are some examples of vaginal probiotics on the market:

- Love Wellness- Good Girl Probiotics

- O Positiv Health URO Vaginal Probiotics

- Metagenics UltraFlora

- Bonafide Clairvee

NOTES

NOTES TO INTRODUCTION

NICE, (2021, June 29). Teach pelvic floor lessons in schools, says guidelines. BBC News.
https://www.bbc.com/news/health-57640558

Subak, L. L., Brubaker, L., Chai, T. C., Creasman, J. M., Diokno, A. C., Goode, P. S., Kraus, S. R., Kusek, J. W., Leng, W. W., Lukacz, E. S., Norton, P., Tennstedt, S., & Urinary Incontinence Treatment Network (2008). High costs of urinary incontinence among women electing surgery to treat stress incontinence. *Obstetrics and Gynecology, 111*(4), 899–907.
https://doi.org/10.1097/AOG.0b013e31816a1e12

Wu, J., Vaughan, C., Goode, P., Redden, T., Burgio, K., Richter, H., and Markland, A. (2014). Prevalence and Trends of Symptomatic Pelvic Floor Disorders in U.S. Women. *Obstetrics and Gynecology*, 123(1): 141-8.
https://www.ncbi.nlm.nih.gov/pmc/articles/PMC3970401/

NOTES TO CHAPTER 1

Gram, M. C. D., & Bø, K. (2020). High level rhythmic gymnasts and urinary incontinence: Prevalence, risk factors, and influence on performance. *Scandinavian journal of medicine & science in sports*, *30*(1), 159–165.
https://doi.org/10.1111/sms.13548

Hallock, J. L., and Handa, V. L. (2016). The Epidemiology of Pelvic Floor Disorders and Childbirth: An Update. *Obstetrics and gynecology clinics of North America, 43*(1), 1–13. https://doi.org/10.1016/j.ogc.2015.10.008

Rortveit, G., Subak, L. L., Thom, D. H., Creasman, J. M., Vittinghoff, E., Van Den Eeden, S. K., and Brown, J. S. (2010). Urinary incontinence, fecal incontinence and pelvic organ prolapse in a population-based, racially diverse cohort: prevalence and risk factors. *Female pelvic medicine & reconstructive surgery, 16*(5), 278–283. https://doi.org/10.1097/SPV.0b013e3181ed3e31

Smith CP. Male chronic pelvic pain: An update. Indian J Urol. 2016 Jan-Mar;32(1):34-9

NOTES TO CHAPTER 2

Anderson, J., Baird, P., Davis, R., Ferreri, S., Knudtson, M., Koraym, A., Waters, V., and Williams, C. (2009). Health benefits of dietary fiber, *Nutrition Reviews, 67*(4):188–205, https://doi.org/10.1111/j.1753-4887.2009.00189.x

Bogaert, G., Stein, R., Undre, S., Nijman, R. J. M., Quadackers, J., 't Hoen, L., Kocvara, R., Silay, S., Tekgul, S., Radmayr, C., & Dogan, H. S. (2020). Practical recommendations of the EAU-ESPU guidelines committee for monosymptomatic enuresis-Bedwetting. Neurourology and urodynamics, 39(2), 489–497. https://doi.org/10.1002/nau.24239

Brown, L., Rosner, B., Willett, W., and Sacks, F. (1999). Cholesterol-lowering effects of dietary fiber: a meta-analysis, *The American Journal of Clinical Nutrition, 69*(1): 30–42, https://doi.org/10.1093/ajcn/69.1.30

Chung, B., Parekh, U., and Sellin, J. (1999). The Effect of increased fluid intake on stool output in normal healthy volunteers. *J Clin Gastroenterol. 28*: 29–32

Grandjean, AC, Reimers KJ, Bannick, KE, and Haven, MC. (2000). The effect of caffeinated, non-caffeinated, caloric, and non-caloric beverages on hydration. *Journal Am Coll Nutr 19*: 591–600

Kranz, S., Brauchla, M., Slavin, J., and Miller, K. (2012). What Do We Know about Dietary Fiber Intake in Children and Health? The Effects of Fiber Intake on Constipation, Obesity, and Diabetes in Children. *Advances in Nutrition, 3*(1): 47–53, https://doi.org/10.3945/an.111.001362

Litwin, M., Melmed, G. and Nakazon, T. (2001) 'LIFE AFTER RADICAL PROSTATECTOMY: A LONGITUDINAL STUDY', The Journal of Urology, 166(2), pp. 587–592. doi:https://doi.org/10.1016/S0022-5347(05)65989-7.

Miketinas, D., Bray, G., Beyl, R., Ryan, D., Sacks, F., and Champagne, C. (2019). Fiber Intake Predicts Weight Loss and Dietary Adherence in Adults Consuming Calorie-Restricted Diets: The POUNDS Lost. *The Journal of Nutrition and Disease 149*(10): 1742-1748.

Reynolds, A., Mann, J., Cummings, J., Winter, N., Mete, E., & Morenga, L. (2019). Carbohydrate Quality Human Health Series of Systematic Reviews and Meta-Analyses. *The Lancet,*

393: pp. 434-435

The National Academy of Sciences (2019). Dietary references intakes for water, potassium, sodium, chloride, and sulfate. https://nap.nationalacademies.org/read/10925/chapter/6#102. Accessed on 9/1/2022.

USDA National Nutrient Database for Standard Reference, Legacy Release. U.S. Department of Agriculture, Agricultural Research Service. https://ndb.nal.usda.gov. Accessed Nov. 7, 2018.

U.S. Department of Health and Human Services and U.S. Department of Agriculture. 2015 – 2020 Dietary Guidelines for Americans. 8th Edition. December 2015. Available at https://health.gov/our-work/food-nutrition/previous-dietary-guidelines/2015.

NOTES TO CHAPTER 4

Curillo-Aguirre, C. A., & Gea-Izquierdo, E. (2023). Effectiveness of Pelvic Floor Muscle Training on Quality of Life in Women with Urinary Incontinence: A Systematic Review and Meta-Analysis. Medicina (Kaunas, Lithuania), 59(6), 1004. https://doi.org/10.3390/medicina59061004

NOTES TO CHAPTER 5

Cohen, D., Gonzalez, J., & Goldstein, I. (2016). The Role of Pelvic Floor Muscles in Male Sexual Dysfunction and Pelvic

Pain. *Sexual Medicine Review, 4*(1):53–62, https://doi.org/10.1016/j.sxmr.2015.10.001.

Franco, M., Pena, C., Freitas, L., Lucia, F., Cristine, L., and Ferreira, H. (2021). Pelvic Floor Muscle Training Effect in Sexual Function in Postmenopausal Women: A Randomized Controlled Trial, *The Journal of Sexual Medicine, 18*(7):1236-1244. https://doi.org/10.1016/j.jsxm.2021.05.005.

Kanter, G., Rogers, R.G., Pauls, R.N., Kammerer-Doak, D., and Thakar, R., (2015). A strong pelvic floor is associated with higher rates of sexual activity in women with pelvic floor disorders. *Int Urogynecol J* 26, 991–996. https://doi.org/10.1007/s00192-014-2583-7

Kizilkaya, N., Yalicin, O., and Erkan H. (2003). The effect of pelvic floor training on sexual function of treated patients. *Int Urogynecol J Pelvic Floor Dysfunction, 14*:234–238.

Kolberg-Tennfjord, M., Hilde, G., Stær-Jensen, J., Siafarikas, F., EllstrӧmEngh, M., and Bø, K. (2015). ("Pelvic floor muscle function, vaginal symptoms and symptoms of sexual ...") Effect of postpartum pelvic floor muscle training on vaginal symptoms and sexual dysfunction—secondary analysis of a randomized trial. *Int. Jour. Obstetrics and Gynecology, 123*(4): 634-642

Lowenstein, L., Gruenwald, I., Gartman, I., and Vardi, Y. (2010). Can stronger pelvic muscle floor improve sexual function? *Int Urogynecol J 21*, 553–556. https://doi.org/10.1007/s00192-009-1077-5

Mercier, J., Morin, M., Lemieux, M., Reichetzer, B., Khalifé, S., and Dumoulin, C. (2016). Pelvic floor muscles training to reduce symptoms and signs of vulvovaginal atrophy: a case study. *Journal of Menopause, 23*(7):816-820(5). https://doi.org/10.1097/GME.0000000000000620.

Sartori, D., Kawano, P., Yamamoto, H., Guerra, R., Pajolli, P., and Amaro, J. (2021). Pelvic floor muscle strength is correlated with sexual function. *Journal of Investigative and Clinical Urology, 62*: 79-85. https://doi.org/10.4111/icu.20190248

NOTES TO CHAPTER 6

Beckmann, M., and Garrett, A. (2006). Antenatal perineal massage for reducing perineal trauma. *Cochrane Database System Review 1*: CD005123

Hormone Health Network. "Relaxin | Endocrine Society." Hormone.org, *Endocrine Society*, Nov. 2018, www.hormone.org/your-health-and-hormones/glands-and-hormones-a-to-z/hormones/relaxin.

Magoga et al. (2019). Warm perineal compresses during the second stage of labor for reducing perineal trauma: A meta-analysis. Eur J Obstet Gynecol Reprod Biol. 240: 93-98

Molinet Coll, C., Martínez Franco, E., Altimira Queral, L., Cuadras, D., Amat Tardiu, L., and Parés, D. (2022). Hormonal Influence in Stress Urinary Incontinence During Pregnancy and Postpartum. *Reproductive sciences (Thousand Oaks, Calif.)*, 10.1007/s43032-022-00946-7. Advance online publication. https://doi.org/10.1007/s43032-022-00946-7

Perelmuter, S., Burns, R., Shearer, K., Grant, R., Soogoor, A., Jun, S., Meurer, J. A., Krapf, J., & Rubin, R. (2024). Genitourinary syndrome of lactation: a new perspective on postpartum and lactation-related genitourinary symptoms. *Sexual medicine reviews*, qeae034. Advance online publication. https://doi.org/10.1093/sxmrev/qeae034

Rajavuori, A., Repo, J. P., Häkkinen, A., Palonen, P., Multanen, J., and Aukee, P. (2021). Maternal risk factors of urinary incontinence during pregnancy and postpartum: A prospective cohort study. European journal of obstetrics & gynecology and reproductive biology: X, 13, 100138.https://doi.org/10.1016/j.eurox.2021.100138

NOTES TO CHAPTER 7

Kolodynska, G., Zalewski, M., and Rozek-Piechura, K. (2019). Urinary incontinence in postmenopausal women-causes, symptoms, treatment. *Menopause Review, 18*(1):46-50

Mercier, J., Morin, M., Zaki, D., Reichetzer, B., Lemieux, M., Khalifé, S., and Dumoulin, C. (2019). Pelvic floor muscle training as a treatment for genitourinary syndrome of menopause: A single-arm feasibility study. *Maturitas, 125*:57-62. https://doi.org/10.1016/j.maturitas.2019.03.002.

Nazarpour, S., Simbar, M., Majd, A., and Tehrani, F. (2018). Beneficial effects of pelvic floor muscle exercises on sexual function among postmenopausal women: a randomized clinical trial. *Sexual Health 15*(5) 396-402 https://doi.org/10.1071/SH17203

NOTES TO CHAPTER 8

Basair-Castillo, C., Carrasco-Portino, M., Valenzuela-Peters, R., Orellana-Gaete, L., Viveros-Allende, V., and Ruiz-Cantero, M. (2022). Effect of conservative treatment of pelvic floor dysfunction in women: an umbrella review. *Int. Journal of Gynecology and Obstetrics.* https://doi.org/10.1002/ijgo.14172

Boyd, S., Subramanian, D., Propst, K., O'Sullivan, D., & Tulikangas, P. (2021). Pelvic organ prolapse severity and genital hiatus size with long-term pessary use. *Female Pelvic Medicine & Reconstructive Surgery, 27*(2) - p e360-e362 DOI: 10.1097/SPV.0000000000000937

Cheung, R., Lee, J., Lee, L., Chung, T., and Chan, S. (2016). Vaginal pessary in women with symptomatic pelvic organ prolapse. *Obstetrics & Gynecology, 128*(1):73-80(8)

Daman-Van Beek Z, Teunissen D, Dekker JH, et al. (2016). Practice guidelines 'urinary incontinence in women' from the Dutch College of General Practitioners. *Ned Tijdschr Geneeskd.,* 160. D674.

Jarvis, S. K., Hallam, T. K., Lujic, S., Abbott, J. A., & Vancaillie, T. G. (2005). Perioperative physiotherapy improves outcomes for women undergoing incontinence and or prolapse surgery: results of a randomized controlled trial. *The Australian & New Zealand Journal of Obstetrics &Gynecology, 45*(4), 300–303. https://doi.org/10.1111/j.1479-828X.2005.00415.x

Kolodynska, G., Zalewski, M., and Rozek-Piechura, K.

(2019). Urinary incontinence in postmenopausal women-causes, symptoms, treatment. *Menopause Review, 18*(1):46-50

Syan, R. and Brucker, B. (2016). Guideline of guidelines: urinary incontinence. *British Journal of Urology, 117*: 20-33.

Thompson, J.A., O'Sullivan, P.B., Briffa, N.K., & Neumann, P. (2006). Assessment of voluntary pelvic floor muscle contraction in continent and incontinent women using transperineal ultrasound, manual muscle testing, and vaginal squeeze pressure measurements. *Int. Urogynecology Journal, pp. 17*, 624–630

Van der Vaart, L., Vollebregt, A., Milani, A., Largo-Janseen, A., Duijnhoven, R., Roovers, J., and Van der Vaart, C. (2022). Pessary or surgery for a symptomatic pelvic organ prolapse: the PEOPLE study, a multicentre prospective cohort study. *BJOG, 129*(5):820-829.

Weber-Rajek, M., Straczynska, A., Strojek, K., Piekorz, Z., Pilarska, B., Podgorica, M., Sobieralska-Michalak, K., and Goch, A., and Radziminska, A. (2020). Assessment of the Effectiveness of Pelvic Floor Muscle Training (PFMT) and Extracorporeal Magnetic Innervation (ExMI) in Treatment of Stress Urinary Incontinence in Women: A Randomized Controlled Trial. *BioMed Res. Int.* 1019872

NOTES TO APPENDIX

Dos Santos, C. C. M., Uggioni, M. L. R., Colonetti, T., Colonetti, L., Grande, A. J., & Da Rosa, M. I. (2021). Hyaluronic Acid in Postmenopause Vaginal Atrophy: A

Systematic Review. *The journal of sexual medicine, 18*(1), 156–166. https://doi.org/10.1016/j.jsxm.2020.10.016

Gupta, V., Mastromarino, P., & Garg, R. (2024). Effectiveness of Prophylactic Oral and/or Vaginal Probiotic Supplementation in the Prevention of Recurrent Urinary Tract Infections: A Randomized, Double-Blind, Placebo-Controlled Trial. *Clinical infectious diseases: an official publication of the Infectious Diseases Society of America, 78*(5), 1154–1161. https://doi.org/10.1093/cid/ciad766

ABOUT THE AUTHOR

I have been a Physical Therapist since 1992 and have successfully helped thousands of patients. I offer the highest standard of patient care, integrity, devotion, and compassion. My goal is to help my patients regain function and improve their overall quality of life. I hope you enjoyed and learned something from this book.

Sincerely,

Natalie

Dr. Natalie Padveen, PT, DPT

Leak No More

Leak No More

Leak No More

Printed in Great Britain
by Amazon